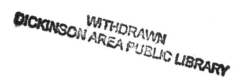
Blood Pressure

Step By Step Guide And Proven Recipes To Lower Your Blood Pressure Without Any Medication

Table Of Content

Introduction

Hypertension – or high blood pressure – is one of the world's deadliest medical conditions. For one, it's a very covert assassin – one that builds up slowly over time without people knowing it. Another reason why it's such a deadly condition is that it increases the risks for other serious medical conditions such as heart attacks, renal failure, stroke, and aneurysms. Lastly, it's a very deadly medical condition because it's often the result of something that most people find hard to control – diet. Now more than ever, hypertension continues to afflict and affect millions and millions of people the world over.

But hypertension isn't an unbeatable foe. In fact, hypertension is a medical condition that can be easily prevented and the chances of being able to successfully bring down one's blood pressure are high. As such, hypertension isn't necessarily a death sentence. The battle against it can be won.

And that's what this book's about – winning the battle against hypertension or high blood pressure. You will read about the 3 foundations of successful and natural management of hypertension (without expensive maintenance medicines) and practical ways on how to do well in each. As a bonus, I've included 9 deliciously healthy and easy to prepare recipes that will help you hit the ground running when it comes to hypertension management. Who says living healthy can't be fun and delicious?

So if you're ready, turn the page and let's begin!

Bonus: FREE Report Reveals The Secrets To Lose Weight

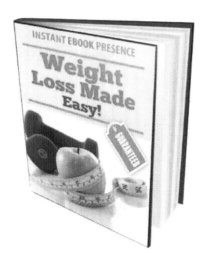

Weight loss doesn't happen from dieting only. Diets are short term solutions to shed extra weight. Diets do not work in the long term because people hate being on a diet (it's ok, you can admit that here). The only long term solution for permanent weight loss is to create new eating habits. This doesn't mean that chocolate will never pass your lips again, but it does mean looking after yourself and watching what you eat...

You can lose weight when you have the right reasons and motivation, and a part of this guide is to help you to find the motivation you need to change your weight...

Click Here to Get This Guid For FREE

Chapter 1: Blood Pressure 101

High blood pressure – also known as hypertension – is one of the most common medical conditions in the world today. In the United States alone, there are about 60 million who suffer from the condition. So what makes for high blood pressure how do you know if you have it?

Basically, blood pressure refers to how much force is pressed or exerted on the artery's wall as blood is pumped through it to the rest of the body. Whenever your heart beats, it can pump up to 3 ounces of blood through your body's main arteries that lead to organs. If you want a better picture of how that looks like, think of a garden hose to which several garden sprinklers are attached. When water pressure is too low, you'll notice that the hose is rather soft and not enough water flows through it to the plants around the garden. On the other hand, the hose can be so hard if the water pressure's too strong or high. And if the garden hose is made from very poor quality materials, it's possible for it to burst or have leakages.

In essence, that's what your blood pressure is all about. Substitute your heart for the faucet or tap, the arteries for the garden hose, blood for water, and the garden's plants to your body's cells. If your heart pumps blood so strongly that the pressure inside the arteries is so high, it can lead to serious medical conditions.

Going back to the garden hose analogy, water pressure from the tap is usually not too strong to increase the water pressure inside the garden hose. Often times, what causes water pressure to increase substantially at any points in the hose are obstructions, whether its sharp bending of the hose, stepping on it, or something stuck inside – blocking the flow of water. In some cases though, it can be a result of too much water pressure too. It's the same with your blood pressure. In most cases, the arteries are obstructed leading to high blood pressure. In some cases too, it's about sheer volume of blood.

Measuring blood pressure

So how do you measure your blood pressure? Regardless if you're using a manual or digital blood pressure monitoring device called a sphygmomanometer, sphygmo for short, two numbers are relevant: the systole and the diastole. The systole represents the pressure of blood flowing out of the heart while the diastole represents the pressure of blood flowing back into it. In other words, blood pressure – as a measurement – is determined by the heart both working (systole) and resting (diastole).

When reading blood pressure measurements, such as 110 mmHg over 70 mmHg, it means that your heart's beating measure and the peak pressure your arteries are subject to at the time of blood pressure measurement is 110 millimeters of mercury (mmHg) and that the pressure in between heart beats – the lowest pressure applied to your arteries – is 70 mmHg.

Normal blood pressure isn't a one-size fits all measurement. "Normal" means different levels for different people depending on age, gender, and physical activity, among other things. Incidentally, the reason why you see sphygmoes being attached to the upper arm when taking blood pressure measurements is because it's where a very good representative artery can be easily accessed. While there's another one on your neck, it just looks plain weird – and somewhat dangerous – to attach the sphygmo on your neck and get chocked to death in the name of monitoring your blood pressure.

So how is your blood pressure measured or taken? Here are the steps:

- With your arm at the same level as your heart – straight or bent at the elbows is fine – wrap the sphygmo's cuff around your upper arm at about an inch above your elbow. Find your brachial arterial pulse and put a stethoscope there and put the two other ends in your ear to listen to your pulse later. If you're using a digital sphygmo, just follow the instructions on the user's manual and you should be fine. Otherwise, proceed.

- Close the valve of the bulb that's squeezed to pump air into the cuff that's already wrapped around your upper arm. Doing so will make sure that the cuff will be inflated later on.

- Quickly squeeze the bulb several times to inflate the cuff and watch the sphygmometer's measurement's – it can either be a column of mercury or a dial – measure until it reaches about 200mmHg. At which point, stop squeezing the bulb and slightly open the valve to let air out at a relatively slow pace.

- As the cuff deflates, listen to the sound of your pulse using the stethoscope while looking at the sphygmo's measurement. When you first hear a pulse, note at which point of the measurement that happened. That would be your top or systolic pressure, e.g., 120mmHg.

- Continue listening to you pulse and monitoring the measurement. The point or measurement at which the pulse is last heard is your lower or diastolic pressure, e.g., 85mmHg. That gives you your blood pressure, e.g., 120mmHG/85mmHg.

Back in the day, if you had a blood pressure of 140/90, yours would still be considered "normal", albeit on the upper limit of the spectrum. These days however, it's no longer the norm. According to experts, a blood pressure of 120/80 is considered normal. Pre hypertensive blood pressure is one with a systolic pressure of up to 139mmHg and a diastolic pressure of up to 89mmHg. You're already considered hypertensive if your systolic blood pressure is at 140mmHg or higher and your diastolic pressure is 90 mmHg or higher.

Take note, however, that those are measurements aren't a one-time big time indicator. What do I mean by this? For one, just because you measured your blood pressure now and it read 135/85 doesn't mean you're already pre-hypertensive. An elevated blood pressure isn't necessarily a sign of hypertension because it may be that your pressure went up because you saw a very hot woman (or man, as the case maybe) just as you were about to measure your blood pressure. It can also be that you're suffering from a really bad case of migraine, which can also temporarily increase your blood pressure.

Another thing about being considered pre-hypertensive or hypertensive is the consistency of the measurement. If you measure your blood pressure thrice a day (morning, noon and night) and your average blood pressure is above 135/85 for several days, i.e., it's persistent, then you may possibly be suffering from hypertension already.

So if you're average blood pressure is persistently elevated even if you're rested and aren't suffering from any emotional, mental or physical discomfort, then it's time to consult with your doctor already.

Kinds Of Hypertension

8

When it comes to high blood pressure, there are 3 classifications: primary (also called essential), secondary (also called non-essential), or isolated systolic. The primary type of hypertension is one for which there is no actual reason or cause. The secondary type of hypertension is the type that has some identifiable and manageable trigger or case like specific types of medicines or pregnancy (preeclampsia). The isolated systolic is the kind of hypertension is the type where the systolic blood pressure is elevated during heartbeats but normalizes in between beats.

Chapter 2: Health Risks

Hypertension is often referred to as a "silent killer' considering that it can subtly cause significant damage to you body over time and by the time symptoms of such damages appear, it's often too late. If left unmanaged, hypertension can cause poor life quality, a permanent disability, or a fatal case of heart attack. About 50% of those who are afflicted with this medical condition who don't manage or have it treated tend to die due to heart ailments such as ischemic heart disease because blood flow is severely affected and about 30% suffer from fatal strokes.

When your blood pressure is persistently high, it means that your blood vessels' walls are under a lot of force, which can also affect your brain, eyes, kidneys, and heart. And when it comes to strokes, hypertension is the primary reason for most cases of such, regardless if it's the direct or indirect reason. Hypertension's also a key risk factor for renal disease and failure, and heart attacks.

Fortunately, being diagnosed with hypertension doesn't have to be a death sentence. With regular treatment and some changes in lifestyle, hypertension can be managed well and minimize the risks for potentially fatal complications. But if left untreated or unmanaged, the following health risks become much, much higher.

Arterial Damage

When your arteries are elastic, strong and flexible, they're healthy. And when they're healthy, the inner linings allow for the free and smooth flow of blood through them on the way to supplying oxygen and nutrients to key tissues and organs of your body.

When you suffer from hypertension, your blood flow's pressure on your arteries tend to increase over time, which can lead to your arteries' pathways becoming narrower and narrower, as well as getting damaged. Hypertension can cause damage to the cells that comprise your arteries lining. And as dietary fat accumulates inside your blood stream when you have a consistently high-fat diet, they can significantly reduce your arteries' elasticity and eventually, blood flow is impeded.

Hypertension can also cause weakened portions of your arteries to grow or expand and create an aneurysm or a bulge. The danger lies in the risk of such aneurysms rupturing and result in fatal internal hemorrhaging or bleeding. Aneurysms can manifest in just about any artery anywhere in the body but the most prevalent cases happen in the aorta, the body's biggest artery.

Cardio Damage

Unmanaged hypertension can lead to cardio or heart damage in several ways. First, it can lead to a condition known as coronary heart disease, which is affliction of the arteries that bring blood to the heart. Free movement of blood through the coronary artery is impeded by arteries that have narrowed down as a result of this condition. One of the symptoms of this condition is chest pain, arrhythmias (irregular heart beat) or worse, heart attack.

Hypertension can also damage the heart by enlarging its left ventricle. Consistently high blood pressure tends to makes it much harder to pump blood throughout your body, which is the function of the left ventricle. When it works much harder over extended periods of time, it can become thick or stiff, which significantly reduces its ability to supply the rest of your body with blood. This in turn significantly raises your risks for a sudden cardiac arrest, heart failure, and heart attack.

Lastly, hypertension can cause your heart to just flat out fail on you. Consistently high blood pressure – if unmanaged – can over time strain your muscle to the point where it can become weaker and less efficient. When this continues, it'll simply tire out and just...fail!

Brain Damage

Your brain is very similar to your heart in that it's highly dependent on getting enough nourishment through your blood for optimal health and performance. Hypertension can get in the way via TIAs or transient ischemic attacks, also referred to as "mini-strokes". This is a momentary disturbance in the amount of blood that flows to the brain, which is oftentimes a result of blood clots or atherosclerosis – both may be caused by hypertension. TIAs are very accurate indicators of a potential full-blown stroke that's waiting to happen.

Speaking of such, a stroke happens when a section of your brain isn't able to get enough nutrients and oxygen (via blood), which result in the death of specific brain cells. Unmanaged hypertension may lead to stroke by making the blood vessels in your brain weak, and cause your brains blood vessels to leak or worse, rupture. Hypertension can also lead to blood clotting in your brain's arteries, which can lead to blood flow blockage and a full-blown stroke.

Dementia is another potential effect of hypertension. This condition is one that causes difficulties when it comes to reasoning, thinking, speaking, moving, seeing, and remembering. Dementia is caused by many things, which includes blockage or reduced blood flow going to the brain.

Strokes can also be the reason for dementia. And in both causes, hypertension is a potential suspect.

Hypertension can also cause a mental condition called mild cognitive impairment, which may be considered as a halfway point from changes in the ability to understand and remember towards more serious conditions such as Alzheimer's disease. Hypertension can cause disruptions in blood flow to the brain that can lead to this mental condition via arterial damage.

Kidney Damage

Speaking of renal failure, how does hypertension cause it? It's because the kidney is somewhat responsible for regulating its own blood flow in pretty much the same way the brain does to its own. When blood pressure is elevated, it changes the way the kidneys regulate its blood flow. Over time, this can lead to damages in the small blood vessels of the kidney, leads to disruption in blood flow, and eventually damage to the organ itself. It's worse for people who also suffer from diabetes because sugar can negatively affect how the efficiency at which the kidneys are able to filter what needs to be filtered.

Hypertension can lead to kidney failure as it damages the glomeruli (tiny blood vessels within your kidneys) as well as the large arteries through which blood flows to it. Damage to just one of them can significantly affect your kidneys' ability to filter out waste from your blood. If left unmanaged, it may come to a point where your kidneys eventually fail and you'll need to undergo dialysis or worse, kidney transplant.

Kidney scars – also called glomerulsclerosis – is another way by which hypertension can damage your kidneys, if left unmanaged. It's a kind of condition or damage to your kidneys that's brought about by scarring of glomeruli, which are essentially small clusters of blood vessels found inside the kidneys. The function of glomeruli is to filter out the waste and water from your blood and glomerulosclerosis keeps them from normally functioning.

Unmanaged hypertension can also lead to aneurysm in the arteries of the kidneys (renal aneurysm). As mentioned earlier, aneurysms are bumps or bulges on the arteries' walls. A possible cause of this is weakening and damaging of the arterial walls due to atherosclerosis. Unmanaged hypertension can lead to enlargement and bulging of renal arteries, which can rupture and lead to fatal renal hemorrhaging.

Eye Damage

Unmanaged hypertension can damage the blood vessels inside your eyes, a condition called retinopathy. This leads to hemorrhaging inside the eyes, which can blur your vision or worse, cause blindness. Greater is your risk if aside from hypertensive, you're also diabetic.

Unmanaged hypertension can also cause buildup of fluids under your retina, a condition referred to as choroidopathy. This is caused by blood vessels under the retina that have leaks. Choroidopathy – or scars resulting from it – may lead to impaired vision.

Lastly, unmanaged hypertension may damage your eyes optic nerves, a condition called optic neuropathy. In this condition, damage is brought about by blood flow that's blocked, which can lead to retinal hemorrhaging or worse, blindness.

Poor Sexual Performance

Particularly for men, unmanaged hypertension may lead to significantly less ability to attain and maintain good erections –

a.k.a. erectile dysfunction – once they turn 50 years old. This is because erections are dependent on the ability of blood to flow within the penile blood vessels and unmanaged hypertension can lead to the narrowing and damaging of these vessels that can impede the all-important penile blood flow.

But it's not always the men who can suffer from poor sexual performance due to unmanaged hypertension – women can suffer from it too. How? High blood pressure minimizes blood flow to the vagina, which may minimize their ability to get aroused and lubricated. When these happen, it's hard for women to enjoy sex and it's practically impossible to achieve orgasm.

Bone Loss

Osteoporosis is another potential health risk associated with unmanaged hypertension. This is because high blood pressure can lead to higher amounts of calcium being excreted from your body via urination. And the more calcium leaks out of your body, the less of it goes to your bones. When your bones get less and less calcium over extended periods of time, osteoporosis may be the result. The risk is actually much higher in women than men.

Sleep Apnea

More than just really loud snoring, sleep apnea is a medical condition that disrupts breathing during sleep due to the relaxation of the throat. Its connection with hypertension? Most people with unmanaged hypertension suffer from sleep apnea. Some even believe that hypertension itself causes sleep apnea. Worse, poor quality and quantity of sleep due to sleep apnea can exacerbate hypertension, kind of like the chicken-or-the-egg conundrum.

Sudden Hypertension Emergencies

Normally, the health damage hypertension causes happens gradually over a long period of time. However, there are instances where blood pressure can swiftly and greatly increase so much so that it becomes a medical emergency that necessitates immediate medical attention. Such a sudden rise in blood pressure can lead to chest pains, pregnancy complications (e.g., eclampsia or preeclampsia), heart attacks, loss of memory, sudden changes in personality, becoming very irritable, problems concentrating, stroke, shortness of breath due to build up of fluid in the longs as a result of sudden impairment in the heart's ability to pump blood (pulmonary edema), and sudden failure of the kidneys.

Chapter 3: Risk Factors

Different factors determine your propensity for becoming hypertensive. One of them is age, which is pretty much a risk factor for most medical conditions. When it comes to men, hypertension is more common when they turn 45 years old. For women, their risk becomes higher once they reach 65 or when they reach menopause.

Certain races of people – probably due to genetic makeup – tend to be at higher risk for hypertension than others. In the United States for example, hypertension is more common among African-Americans than the White Americans. It's not surprising to note that hypertension-related medical conditions such as kidney failure, heart attack, and stroke are more common in African-Americans as well.

Hypertension is also considered to be largely genetic. It doesn't necessarily mean that if your folks or grandparents are hypertensive, you're a shoo-in for the same. Your genes however, can make it much easier for you to become hypertensive compared to others whose family history precludes hypertension. As such, you'll have to take greater care of your health than the average person if indeed this medical condition runs in the family.

Your bodyweight – believe it or not – is another risk factor for hypertension. Why? It's because the higher your body weight, the more there is of you that needs nutrients and oxygen. When the volume of blood needed to bring the right amounts of nutrients and oxygen all over your body increases, so does the pressure needed to ensure adequate blood flow. Fortunately, this is one major risk factor that you can greatly control or manage.

Living a sedentary lifestyle is another key risk factor in developing hypertension. It's because the less active you are physically, the higher your heart rate tends to be. And when your heart rate is constantly elevated, your heart needs to work much harder with every contraction, which significantly increases the amount of pressure exerted on your arteries, i.e., blood pressure. It also doesn't help that being sedentary significantly increases your risks for obesity, which is another major hypertension factor.

The chemicals found in tobacco, regardless if you're smoking or just chewing it, can damage your arterial walls' lining, aside from the fact that smoking or chewing tobacco leads to a temporary rise in your blood pressure. When smoking or chewing tobacco becomes a persistent habit, your temporary elevated blood pressure becomes a chronic one that may increase even more over time. And don't think non-smokers aren't spared – second hand smoke is just as deadly, if not deadlier.

Another major factor for developing hypertension is diet. Fortunately, it's a factor that you have total control over. In particular, the excess amount of sodium you regularly consume can lead to hypertension because sodium makes your body retain more water than what's necessary. Water retention raises blood pressure and so reducing sodium in your diet is key to warding off or managing hypertension.

Another diet related risk factor for hypertension are potassium and Vitamin D deficiencies. Lack of potassium may lead to excess retention of sodium and Vitamin D deficiency can get in the way of your kidneys producing a helpful enzyme for regulating blood pressure. Make sure to get enough of these nutrients in your daily diet.

If you're a heavy alcohol drinker or an alcoholic, I'm sorry to say but excessive drinking won't just damage your liver but can also lead to hypertension, which can result in other serious medical conditions such as heart disease. The good news is you don't have to go cold turkey – you just need to drink in moderation, which are no more than 2 servings and 1 serving daily for men and women, respectively. One serving is about 12 ounces your favorite beer, 1 ½ ounces of hard liquor (80-proof), and 5 ounces of wine.

Lastly, lifestyle is one of the biggest risk factors for hypertension. In particular, stress levels can wreak havoc on your blood pressure if not managed well. If you tend to cope with stress through smoking, binge eating, or drinking alcohol, then you're increasing your risk for hypertension even more!

Chapter 4: Nutritional Approach To Lowering Blood Pressure

When it comes to managing hypertension, the single biggest factor is nutrition or diet. The saying "garbage in, garbage out" is certainly applicable to eating and managing hypertension. If you eat poorly, your health becomes poor as well, e.g., hypertension.

There are many approaches to eating for managing and bringing down blood pressure. And in the last decade or so, one approach has been garnering a lot of attention and accolades simply because it works well when it comes to the battle to control or alleviate hypertension – the DASH diet.

Though the acronyms spell a word that denotes speed of eating, it's anything but. The letters in the acronym stand for Dietary Approaches To Stop Hypertension. As you can see, it's really a diet or a nutritional approach to addressing hypertension.

You may be tempted to think of the DASH diet as another one of those popular starvation, quick weight loss fad diets that you get on for a couple of weeks or months and get off when things become boring or inconvenient. Far from it, the diet is a lifestyle change, i.e., it's a lifelong commitment to eating the right foods in order to bring your blood pressure down to normal.

One thing that distinguishes the DASH diet is its low sodium content. Remember how sodium affects your blood pressure? It's the reason why you will be cutting back down on your foods' sodium content in the DASH diet.

But more than just a low sodium diet, it's one that also rich in key nutrients that, when combined with reduced sodium, can greatly contribute to the ability to bring down high blood pressure. It doesn't hurt that given the right recipes, which I'll provide later on, it can be very delicious one as well!

Within the first few weeks of getting into it, it's possible to bring down your blood pressure by several points. And if you faithfully continue with it, you may even see your blood pressure go down by up to 14 points. And when that happens, it's not just your blood pressure that goes down – so do your other blood pressure-related health risks.

But wait, there's more! A potential and desirable side effect of the diet is also weight loss, which also lowers your risk for obesity-related medical conditions such as diabetes, heart attacks, specific types of cancers, stroke, and osteoporosis. If that's not enough to make you want to do the DASH diet, I don't know what will.

Sodium Content

When it comes to helping your body function normally and stay healthy, sodium is important. Available mostly in salt, sodium allows your body to get the right amounts of electrolytes, which are crucial for your body when it comes to specific functions that require the transmittal of electrical impulses. How? By helping your body retain enough water for such processes or functions, which is also a key determinant of blood pressure.

Aside from helping your body perform functions that require electrical impulses, it also helps you delay or even avoid muscle cramps. Extreme endurance athletes such as ultra-marathoners and triathletes bring salt-sticks or saline solutions on the road during competitions because cramps can spell the difference between finishing and not finishing at all.

To function normally, your body needs on average about 500 milligrams of sodium daily. Unfortunately, many people's diets today tend to overdo the sodium content – reaching up to as much as 10 times more than the requirement or about 5,000 milligrams daily! Is it any wonder then, that more and more people are afflicted with hypertension today than ever before? If going overboard by 3 times is bad enough, what more 10 times?

Normally, your body gets rid of excess amounts of sodium in your blood through the process of urination. But your kidneys are also limited in their ability to do so such that if the amount of sodium in your blood is excessively very high, then your kidneys may not be able to filter all of the excess sodium from your blood. When that happens, the excess amounts of sodium ends up staying in your blood. Here's where it gets interesting.

Do you remember out discussion earlier about how sodium is important for water retention? Because you have so much sodium in your blood, it draws water into your blood stream resulting in swelling of blood volume excessively above the normal. When the volume of your blood is excessively high, the harder your heart needs to work much harder to keep it flowing throughout your body. And guess what? Blood pressure rises as a result of that hard work.

There are 2 benchmarks or standards by which "normal" sodium consumption is observed – at least in the United States: The American Heart Association and the Dietary Guidelines For Americans benchmarks. Under the American Heart Association guidelines, the limit is 1,500 milligrams daily for adults. Under the Dietary Guidelines For Americans benchmark, the maximum amount is 2,300 milligrams. So which one do you follow under the DASH diet?

Well, it depends on your hypertension management goals. If your not yet hypertensive and your goal is to simply minimize your risks for becoming hypertensive, then you can follow the Dietary Guidelines For Americans' maximum daily limit of 2,300 milligrams – the standard version of the DASH diet. If you're already hypertensive, then your goal is obviously to bring your blood pressure down, which means the applicable maximum daily limit for you is the American Heart Association limit of 1,500 milligrams daily – the lower sodium version of the DASH diet.

DASH Eating

Whether you choose the lower sodium or standard version of the DASH diet, you will be eating healthy amounts of vegetables, grains, fruits, and low-fat dairy products. The diet also lets you enjoy some fish, poultry, and legumes. A couple of times weekly, you also get to enjoy small amounts of red meat, fats, sweets, nuts, and seeds. Aside from being low in sodium, the diet is also low in total and saturated fats, as well as cholesterol as these also considered key hypertension factors.

As with other calories, calories also count in the diet. Specifically, daily caloric consumption is limited to more or less 2,000 calories. The amount of food you will eat will also determine your success – or failure – in managing hypertension.

More than just quantity, you will also need to eat the right kinds of foods under the DASH diet. These include:

- Alcohol And Caffeine: Your blood pressure may rise with alcohol and caffeine consumption. While no solid scientific evidence links caffeine consumption with hypertension, it's a well-known scientific fact that caffeine – especially lots of it – can result in spikes in your heart rate and consequently, blood pressure, although it's short-lived. But if you're already hypertensive, better to be safe than sorry and ditch it altogether. But if you really can't resist the taste of coffee, go for decaf as a safe alternative. The Dietary Guidelines For Americans limits alcohol consumption to a maximum of 2 servings for men and a serving for women everyday. Still, I highly recommend ditching it altogether considering they really don't offer any health benefit and that they increase your risks for hypertension.

- Dairy Products: While many dairy products such as milk, yogurt, and cheese are chock full of calcium, Vitamin D, and protein, there's a risk of consuming excess amounts of saturated fats – not DASH diet friendly – if you choose wrongly. The solution: Low-fat dairy products! You can eat as much as 3 servings daily, where a serving may be a cup of skimmed (1%) milk, 1 ½ ounces of partially skimmed cheese, or a cup of yogurt.

- Dietary Fats And Oil: No diet worth its salt will take dietary fat out of the equation. Why? It's because dietary fat enables you body to utilize key fat-soluble vitamins and helps strengthen your immune system. The issue is the same as with sweets: moderation. Too much any good thing eventually becomes bad because it increases your health risks.   And when it comes to "moderation", the DASH diet allows you to get as much as 30% of your daily calories from dietary fat – particularly from monounsaturated fat (the good fat).   As far as servings go, you can have as much as 3 servings daily where a serving may be 2 tablespoons of salad dressing, 1 teaspoon of virgin coconut oil, 1 tablespoon of mayonnaise, or 1 teaspoon of soft margarine. Just make sure to keep clear of saturated and trans fats – the evil fats – that you can usually find in most highly processed treats like baked pastries, French fries, and most crackers. Again, make sure you check the labels to avoid "accidentally" gorging on unhealthy and excessive amounts of dietary fat.

- Fruits: Fruits are an integral part of the DASH diet because they contain generous amounts of several key nutrients: dietary fiber, potassium, and magnesium. Even better, they are generally low in fat, with the exception of coconut and avocado. Fruits can give you a lot of culinary variety under the diet as these can be eaten on their own as snacks, or used as garnishing for your other meals. Under the diet, you can eat as much as 5 servings everyday, where a serving may be ½ cup of fruits, a medium-sized fruit, or up to 4 ounces of freshly squeezed fruit juice or unsweetened canned fruit juice (not juice drinks, which aren't natural). When it comes to citrus fruits and their juices, keep in mind that they can potentially alter the efficacy of specific types of medicines. So if you're the type who loves citrus fruits like grapefruit and would like to make them part of your DASH diet and you're taking maintenance medicines, ask your doctor first if they have the potential to interact with them.

- Lean Meats, Fish, And Poultry: When it comes to getting enough iron, zinc, protein, and B vitamins, the best source for such are red meat (lean cuts). Under the DASH diet however, maximum daily consumption is just 6 ounces. For poultry, limit consumption to the breast part only sans the skin because the skin has high fat content and the breast meat is one of the best sources of lean protein. You can further minimize fat content by baking, broiling, roasting or grilling instead of frying. And when it comes to eating fish, it's best to prioritize those that contain generous amounts of omega-3 fatty acids such as salmon, herring and tuna, which can help bring cholesterol levels down. For fish, you can eat up to 6 servings daily.

- Nuts, Legumes, And Seeds: You can get a lot of magnesium, potassium, and protein from almonds, kidney beans, lentils, peas, and sunflower seeds. Even better, nuts, legumes and seeds contain high amounts of phytochemicals and dietary fiber. Phytochemicals are very helpful in minimizing risks for cardiovascular diseases and even some particular types of cancers. For these, you can eat as much as 5 servings – not daily but on a weekly basis. This is because these types of foods are packed with so much calories that just a little goes a long way towards weight gain. A serving may be 1/3 cup of nuts, 2 tablespoons of seeds, and ½ cup of cooked beans or peas. When it comes to nuts, I'm happy to note that the fat calories they contain are mostly good fats: monounsaturated fats and omega-3 fatty acids, both of which are good for the heart. Just keep them in moderation to avoid weight gain.

- Sweets: The beautiful thing about the DASH diet is that it's not torture. Yes, you can actually eat sweet under the DASH diet. This is one reason why many people are able to stay on the diet for life – it's not as restrictive as the others. However, it's not a free pass to stuff yourself with the stuff everyday. In particular, you should only eat up to a maximum of 5 servings weekly. A serving may be ½ cup of sorbet, 1 cup of lemonade, or a tablespoon of sugar, jelly, and jam. And when you go for your sweet treats, don't forget the habit of checking out the label to ensure that they're either low or non-fat like graham crackers, jellybeans, hard candy, low-fat cookies, sorbet, and fruit ices. You can use a healthy sugar substitute such as stevia for sugar but I highly recommend sticking to the same maximum weekly servings. Why? While it may not contribute much to your caloric intake, it will weaken your willpower, especially when it comes to sweets in general.

–   Veggies: Some of the best under the diet include tomatoes, broccoli, greens, sweet potatoes, and carrots. It's because they're chock full of dietary fiber, key minerals like potassium and magnesium, and vitamins. For veggies, you can eat as much as 5 servings everyday and each serving is about a cup of raw green leafy vegetables or about half a cup of vegetables that are cut up. And when going for veggies that are either canned or frozen, make sure to check that the label says something like "no salt added", "unsalted", or "low sodium".

–   Whole Grains: In particular, you can eat whole wheat grain-based stuff such as whole-wheat pasta and whole-wheat breads, as well as brown rice. Again, be careful to check the label to makes sure it says that the product is 100% made from whole wheat and whole wheat or grain alone. I've seen many bread loaves that say Whole Wheat Bread on the packaging only to find upon checking the label that it's not, e.g., 50% whole-wheat flour and 50% wheat flour. For whole grain products, you can eat as much as 8 servings everyday, where a serving can mean to be a slice of whole-wheat bread, or ½ cup of cooked brown rice or whole-wheat pasta. I highly recommended that bulk of what you'll eat daily under the diet come from whole grains. Why? It's way more satiating of filling, which means your hunger pangs will be minimized. But a more important reason for this is the rich amount of dietary fiber and nutrients that they contain.

Bring The Sodium Down

The foods allowed under the DASH diet are naturally low in sodium, which means that you can lower your blood pressure significantly just by eating the foods allowed under the diet in the right amounts alone. But if you want to up the ante on your sodium reduction efforts, you can bring it down even more through the following practical tips:

- Buying low-sodium, unsalted, and sodium-free packaged foods;

- Choosing to go without salt when cooking brown rice, whole-grain pasta, or hot cereal;

- Spicing up your dishes with salt-free flavorings and spices; and

- Thoroughly rinsing canned foods in order to wash away most of their sodium content.

Major Adjustment

There's always a trade-off between eating healthy and taste. Admittedly, most of the foods you'll be eating under the DASH diet won't be as "tasty" as their very unhealthy counterparts, primarily because of the lower sodium and salt content. So to minimize the "shock" or the feeling of being overwhelmed, I highly recommend that you take baby steps instead of going cold turkey on salty and high sodium-content foods. Rome wasn't built in a day but every hour they were laying bricks, as noted playwright John Heywood. When it comes to fully rolling with the DASH diet, you also need to gradually undo years and years of acclimatization with salty and high-sodium foods and transition into the DASH diet.

Begin by gradually eating more low-sodium foods and lessen the salt content of the foods you eat – in weekly increment and decrements – until you have successfully adjusted to the maximum sodium level recommendation (standard or lower version), according to your goal. As a reminder, if your goal is to just minimize your risk for hypertension, 2,300 milligrams is your maximum daily limit for sodium and if it's to bring down your blood pressure, it's 1,500 milligrams maximum.

Forgive (Yourself) And You Shall Be Forgiven (By Yourself Too)

Before you go and give the DASH diet a committed try, remember that it is a very challenging diet – at least at first. That being said, the best way to destroy your chances of successfully lowering your blood pressure is being very hard or unforgiving of yourself when you "screw" up during the diet, which will inevitably happen. The secret to making the successful transition to the DASH diet and staying there is to learn how to forgive yourself for such screw ups.

There's neither logic nor benefit to beating yourself blind for making mistakes. One, you're human and it's natural to screw up in the beginning, especially with something that's as challenging as the DASH diet. Second, you'll just demoralize yourself into quitting early in the game and continue putting yourself at risk for hypertension and its related medical conditions. As such, forgiving yourself is one of the best ways to motivate yourself under the diet.

Love Yourself

By this, I don't mean to indulge and splurge. What I mean is to reward yourself after each milestone, regardless if it's big or small. Celebrate each and every victory so you'll stay motivated and succeed! By having something to look forward to, you can muster enough strength to take the next step, and the next, and the next until you succeed.

Chapter 5: Recipes

Here's where the nutritional approach to managing hypertension – lowering your blood pressure or simply minimizing your risks for it – come to life. As the saying goes, the proof of the pudding is in the eating. So start eating your way to lower blood pressure with these deliciously easy to prepare DASH diet recipes that will help you launch your anti-hypertension campaign on a deliciously practical note.

<u>Salads</u>

1.) Chicken Salad Grill

Ingredients:

For Preparing The Salad Dressing:

- Cracked Black Pepper;
- Extra-Virgin Olive Oil, 1 Tablespoon;
- Finely Chopped Celery, 1 Tablespoon;
- Finely Chopped Onion, 1 Tablespoon;
- Minced Garlic, 4 cloves; and
- Red Wine Vinegar, ½ Cup.

For Making The Salad:

- 4-Ounce Boneless And Skinless Chicken Breasts, 4 pieces;
- Garlic, 2 cloves;
- Leaf Lettuce, 8 cups;
- Ripe Black Olives, 16 Large Pieces; and

- Sliced And Peeled Navel Oranges, 2 Whole Pieces.

Instructions:

- Prepare the dressing first by mixing all the dressing ingredients in a small mixing bowl until well combined. Put the bowl in the fridge with cover.

- Heat up your grill or broiler and while doing so, take out the grill rack and coat it lightly with cooking spray. When done, place it about 5 inches from the heat.

- Rub the garlic cloves on the chicken breasts and throw the cloves away afterwards. Cook the chicken on the broiler or grill – about 5 minutes per side – until they turn just browned and cooked through. When done, transfer the breasts on a cutting board. Before slicing them into strips, allow them to rest for about 5 minutes.

- Prepare the salad by distributing the orange slices, the olives, and leaf lettuce onto 4 plates (or less, depends on how large you want the servings to be). Top each salad plate with equal amounts of the chicken strips. Drizzle the dressing on the salad, toss, and enjoy!

Total Servings: 4

Nutritional Content Per Serving:

- Calories 237
- Sodium 199 mg
- Added sugars 0 g
- Cholesterol 83 mg
- Dietary fiber 3 g
- Monounsaturated fat 5 g

- Protein 27 g

- Saturated fat 1 g

- Total carbohydrate 12 g

- Total fat 9 g

2.) *Tuna Salad*

Ingredients:

- De-Seeded, De-Spined, And Diced Jalapeno Pepper, 1 Piece;

- Diced Tomato, 1 Medium-Sized Piece;

- Finely Diced Sweet Onion, ½ Piece;

- Lime Juice, 1 Tablespoon;

- Low-Fat Mayonnaise, 2 Tablespoons; and

- Ultra Low Sodium Canned Tuna, 2 cans Of 6 Ounces Each.

Instructions:

- Remove tuna from the water and toss together with all the other ingredients in a medium-sized mixing bowl.

Total Servings: 4

Nutritional Content Per Serving:

- Calories: 127.2

- Sodium: 352.0 mg

- Cholesterol: 27.8 mg

- Dietary Fiber: 0.5 g

- Protein: 22.0 g

- Total Carbs: 3.2 g

- Total Fat: 2.5 g

3.) *Japanese Avocado Salad*

Ingredients

For making the dressing:

- Dijon Mustard, 1 Teaspoon;

- Light Miso, 1 Teaspoon;

- Low-Fat Soya Milk, 1/3 cup;

- Peeled And Minced Ginger, 1 Tablespoon;

- Plain Silken Tofu, 1/3 cup; and

- Reduced Or Low-Sodium Soy Sauce, 1 ½ Teaspoons.

For preparing the salad:

- Baby Lettuce, 12 Ounces;

- Chopped Cilantro, 1 Tablespoon;

- Chopped Fresh Cilantro, 1 Tablespoon;

- Chopped Onion, ¼ Cup;

- Chopped Green Onions, 1 Tablespoon;

- Diagonally Sliced Green Onion, 1 Whole Piece;

- Fresh Lemon Juice, 1 Tablespoon; and

- Peeled And Pitted Avocado, 1 Whole Piece sliced thinly into 12.

Instruction:

- Prepare the dressing by pureeing together the soy milk, tofu, soy sauce, ginger, mustard, and miso using a food processor or a blender until you get a creamy smooth mixture. Pour the mixture on a mixing bowl and mix the green onion and cilantro in until well combined. Leave the mixture in the fridge with cover for a minimum of 1 hour.

- Toss the slices of avocado in lemon juice in a small mixing bowl. This will prevent the slices from turning brown. Set the slices aside after tossing.

- Mix the onions, lettuce, and cilantro together in a big mixing bowl. Toss to combine well.

- Pour about 2/3 of the salad dressing and coat the salad by tossing lightly. Distribute the salad evenly among 6 plates then top each plate with 2 slices of avocados each. Distribute the remaining 1/3 of the salad dressing among the 6 plates to enjoy.

Total Servings: 6

Nutritional Content Per Serving:

- Calories 76
- Sodium 131 mg
- Cholesterol 0 mg
- Dietary fiber 3 g
- Monounsaturated fat 3 g
- Protein 3 g
- Saturated fat 1 g
- Total carbohydrate 7 g

- Total fat 5 g

Side Dishes

1.) Brown Rice Pilaf

Ingredients:

- Canola Oil, 1 ½ Tablespoons;
- Chopped Dried Apricots, ¼ Cup;
- Chopped Pistachios, ¼ Cup;
- Fresh Orange Juice, 3 Tablespoons;
- Grated Orange Zest, ½ Teaspoon;
- Ground Turmeric, ¼ Teaspoon;
- Rinsed And Drained Dark Brown Rice, 1 1/8 Cups;
- Salt, ¾ Teaspoon; and
- Water, 2 Cups.

Instructions:

- Boil together the water, brown rice, turmeric, and ¼ teaspoon of salt in a saucepan in high heat. When it starts to boil, bring heat down to low and simmer with cover for about 45 minutes or until the rice turns tender and has absorbed the water. When done, transfer the rice to a big mixing bowl and let it stay warm.
- Whisk together the remaining salt, canola oil, orange juice and orange zest in a small mixing bowl and when done, pour this mixture on the warm brown rice you've set aside.

- Throw the apricots and nuts in. Coat the mixture by tossing gently before enjoying.

Total Servings: 4

Nutritional Content Per Serving:

- Calories 153

- Sodium 222 mg

- Cholesterol 0 mg

- Dietary fiber 2 g

- Monounsaturated fat 3 g

- Protein 3 g

- Saturated fat 1 g

- Total carbohydrate 24 g

- Total fat 5 g

2.) Broccoli Roast

Ingredients:

- Large Stemmed Broccoli Sliced Into 2-Inch Slices, 8 Cups;

- Olive Oil, 4 Tablespoons – Divided;

- Salt-Free Seasoning, ½ Teaspoon;

- Ground Black Pepper, ¼ Teaspoon;

- Peeled And Minced Garlic, 4 Cloves;

- Crushed Pepper Flakes, ¼ Teaspoon;

Instructions:

- While bringing your oven to 450 degrees Fahrenheit, combine 2 teaspoons of the olive oil with the broccoli in a big mixing bowl by tossing them together. When done, transfer the oiled broccoli on a rimmed baking sheet. Place the sheet inside the preheated oven and allow to bake for up to 15 minutes.

- While the broccoli's baking in the oven, combine the pepper flakes, garlic, and the remaining 2 tablespoons of olive oil. After baking for 15 minutes, drizzle the mixture over the baked broccoli to coat them before baking for another 10 minutes or just until the broccolis become brown. Best enjoyed hot.

Total Servings: 8

Nutritional Content Per Serving:

- Calories: 86
- Sodium: 24 milligrams
- Calcium: 37 milligrams
- Carbohydrate: 5 grams
- Cholesterol: 0 milligrams
- Dietary Fiber: 2 grams
- Fat: 7 grams
- Magnesium: 16 milligrams
- Potassium: 232 milligrams
- Protein: 2 grams
- Saturated Fat: 1 gram
- Sugars: 1 gram

3.) Potato Garlic Mash

Ingredients:

- Gold Potatoes Scrubbed And Cut, 2 Pounds Worth;
- Ground Pepper, ½ Teaspoon;
- Olive Oil, ¼ Cup;
- Peeled Garlic, 6 Cloves; and
- Salt-Free Seasoning, 1 Teaspoon.

Instructions:

- Inside a big saucepan, combine the peeled garlic and potato cuts and boil in water.
- Upon boiling, bring the heat down and cook for 25 minutes more or just until the potatoes turn tender when you poke them with a fork. Remove from heat when done.
- Drain the water from the boiled potatoes except for about ¾ cup of the cooking water. Mix in the all the remaining ingredients with the remaining water and potatoes before mashing the potatoes.

Total Servings: 8

Nutritional Content Per Serving:

- Calories: 145
- Sodium: 7 milligrams
- Calcium: 16 milligrams
- Carbohydrate: 19 grams
- Cholesterol: 0 milligrams

- Dietary Fiber: 2 grams

- Fat: 7 grams

- Magnesium: 26 milligrams

- Potassium: 527 milligrams

- Protein: 2 grams

- Saturated Fat: 1 gram

- Sugars: 1 gram

Main Dishes

1.) Mushroom Burgers

Ingredients:

- Balsamic Vinegar, 1/3 cup;

- Halved Bibb Lettuce Leaves, 2 Pieces;

- Minced Garlic, 1 Clove;

- Olive Oil, 2 Tablespoons;

- Optional: Cayenne Pepper, ¼ Teaspoon;

- Portobello Mushroom Caps, 4 Large Pieces;

- Red Onion, 4 Slices;

- Sugar, 1 Tablespoon;

- Toasted Whole-Wheat Buns, 4 Pieces;

- Tomato, 4 Slices; and

- Water, ½ Cup.

Instructions:

40

- Use a damp cloth to clean the Portobello mushrooms before taking out the stems. Place the large caps on a glass dish with the gill or stem facing upward.

- Prepare the marinade by whisking together the water, vinegar, garlic, sugar, olive oil and cayenne pepper until well combined. Drizzle the Portobello mushrooms with the marinade and refrigerate for 1 hour. Turn the mushrooms once halfway through the marinating process.

- While the mushrooms are in the fridge, heat up your broiler or grill and before placing the rack on the grill, coat it with cooking spray. Place the rack about 6 inches from the grill's heat source.

- On medium heat, broil or grill the Portobello mushrooms for about 5 minutes per side or until tender. To prevent the mushrooms from becoming dry, baste them with the marinade mix while grilling. When done broiling or grilling, transfer the mushrooms to a plate.

- Stuff each of the whole-wheat buns with a mushroom, a slice of tomato, a slice of onion, and ½ leaf of lettuce to enjoy.

Total Servings: 4

Nutritional Content Per Serving:

- Calories 301
- Sodium 163 mg
- Added sugars 3 g
- Cholesterol 0 mg
- Dietary fiber 7 g

- Monounsaturated fat 6 g

- Protein 10 g

- Saturated fat 1 g

- Total carbohydrate 45 g

- Total fat 9 g

- Trans fat 0 g

2.) Salmon Roast

Ingredients:

- 6-Ounce Salmon Fillets, 4 Pieces;

- Lemon Wedges, 4 Pieces;

- Ground Black Pepper;

- Minced Dill, ¼ Cup;

- Peeled And Minced Garlic, 4 Cloves;

Instructions:

- Bring oven to 400 degrees Fahrenheit. While doing so, use a nonstick cooking spray to coat a glass baking dish. Put the salmon fillets inside the coated glass baking dish. On each fillet, squeeze juice from 1 lemon wedge.

- Sprinkle garlic, dill, and ground pepper over the salmon fillets before baking them in the preheated oven for up to 22 minutes or just until the fillets turn opaque at the center.

Total Servings: 4

Nutritional Content Per Serving:

- Calories: 251

- Sodium: 78 milligrams

- Calcium: 36 milligrams

- Carbohydrate: 2 grams

- Cholesterol: 94 milligrams

- Dietary Fiber: less than 1 gram

- Fat: 11 grams

- Magnesium: 53 milligrams

- Potassium: 894 milligrams

- Protein: 34 grams

- Saturated Fat: 2 grams

- Sugars: less than 1 gram

3.) Mexican Mango Pizza

Ingredients

- 12-Inch Homemade Or Packaged Whole-Grain Pizza Crust, 1 Piece;

- Chopped Cilantro, ½ Cup;

- Chopped Green Bell Peppers, 1 Cup;

- Lime Juice, 1 Tablespoon;

- Minced Onion, ½ Cup;

- Peeled, Seeded, And Chopped Mango, ½ Cup; and

- Pineapple Tidbits, ½ Cup.

Instructions:

- Bring your oven to 425 degrees Fahrenheit and while doing so, coat a round baking pan – about 12-inches in diameter – with cooking spray.

- Combine the onions, peppers, pineapple, mango, cilantro, and lime juice in a small mixing bowl then set aside the mango salsa when done.

- Press the whole-wheat crust into the coated baking pan and bake in the pre-heated oven for up to 15 minutes.

- Remove the pizza crust from the oven and spread the salsa all over it before putting it back in the oven to bake for up to 10 minutes more or until the crust turns brown and the toppings become hot.

Total Servings: 4

Nutritional Content Per Serving:

- Calories 250

- Sodium 354 mg

- Added sugars 0 g

- Cholesterol 0 mg

- Dietary fiber 8 g

- Fat 4 g

- Monounsaturated fat 1.5 g

- Protein 8 g

- Saturated fat 1.5 g

- Total carbohydrate 45 g

- Trans fat 0 g

Chapter 6: Physical Approach To Lowering Blood Pressure

While nutrition may be the single biggest factor when it comes to managing blood pressure, there are 2 other important areas that we'll cover that can help you manage and lower your blood pressure. In this chapter, we'll talk about exercising. In the next chapter, we'll talk about lifestyle.

Exercising can significantly help you bring down your blood pressure while helping you manage stress much better (another anti-hypertension bonus), feel better, and enjoy more energy. But before you start on an exercise program – especially if you're already hypertensive – it's best if you check with your doctor first. While the information in this book can be effective in managing or bringing down your blood pressure, it's no substitute for professional medical advice. But since the right exercise will be very helpful in managing your blood pressure, chances are high that your doctor will be very supportive.

When it comes to exercising for managing hypertension, practically anything is possible and you don't have to be limited by the fact that you don't have any fancy exercise equipment at home or that you don't have access to a nearby gym. The general principle that all blood-pressure friendly exercises have in common is the ability to give your heart and lungs just the right amount of exercise to make them stronger and healthier. These include among others jogging, brisk walking, biking, swimming, lifting weights and even doing household chores!

Given the myriad number of ways you can exercise for managing hypertension, how do you know which to perform or get into? You can ask yourself 2 questions to help you figure out which activities you can consistently perform over the long haul: what seems fun to you and whether or not you want to do them alone or with other people.

Types Of Exercises

Generally speaking, there are 3 types of exercises: cardiovascular, resistance, and stretching. Cardiovascular exercises – also called aerobic exercise or aerobics – are the best type when it comes to helping you bring down your blood pressure and ensuring your heart becomes stronger. Generally, these are performed for at least 20 straight minutes per session to have a meaningful effect on your cardiovascular system and includes activities such as dancing, skipping rope, jogging, brisk walking, biking, and swimming.

Resistance training or strength training involves working against a specific form or resistance, such as lifting dumbbells and barbells, with the intention of strengthening and building up the muscles. This type of training or exercise is best for developing muscular, bone, and joint strength.

Stretching exercises are performed with the intention of improving your muscles flexibility, minimizing risks for injuries, and helping you perform certain movements much better.

Exercise Intensity

Intensity refers to how hard you're exercising and the simplest but accurate enough gauge is your breathing. If you're panting and are barely able to catch your breath, you're exercising with too much intensity. If you're able to talk as like you do when you're lying on the couch and talking with your friends without any effort whatsoever, then you're exercising at a very light intensity. The key to achieving cardiovascular health is exercising at a moderate intensity.

How do you know if you're exercising at a moderate intensity? Simple, you can still talk but with just a bit of effort or strain – not too much that you can hardly talk straight. Think of it as a carrying a normal conversation with a little breathing effort.

Intensity is determined by the amount of resistance you're up against and the speed at which you execute the movements. To increase intensity, increase the speed of the movement, the amount of resistance, or both. To decrease intensity, reduce either speed or resistance – or both! When you're running or brisk walking, you can run or walk faster to increase intensity and slower to do the opposite. When lifting weights, increasing the weight lifted is the primary way to increase intensity.

Exercise Duration and Frequency

Next to intensity, you'll need to exercise to make sure you exercise within a specified period of time and a minimum number of times within the week. As mentioned earlier, the minimum duration is 20 straight minutes but ideally, 30 minutes should be your target. Just remember to exercise at moderate intensity all throughout the duration. As for frequency, the best is to do it at least 5 times weekly.

If you have no prior exercising experience whatsoever, don't worry. You can take baby steps by exercising for less than 20 straight minutes, regardless of intensity. The important thing is to get you up and exercising – make it a habit first. Then, you can gradually increase the intensity, duration or both at a pace that's not comfortable but also not strenuous until you're able to exercise for at least 20 straight minutes at moderate intensity.

As you end your exercise session, make it a habit to cool down and stretch. To cool down, spend an extra 2 minutes exercising at light intensity so you can give your heart rate the chance to gradually slow down instead of abruptly dropping back to normal. Also, cooling down allows your body temperature to return to normal gradually instead of abruptly. Both are important if you're hypertensive.

Safety

Generally speaking, exercising at moderate intensity may be considered safe, unless you have a debilitating illness already such as cancer or are suffering from paralysis in some parts of your body due to stroke. As a general guideline, it's still best to ask your doctor for clearance to engage in moderate intensity exercises 5 times a week for at least 20 minutes each session. Better safe than sorry.

The key to exercise safety is warming up and cooling down before and after your exercise sessions, keeping intensity moderate (avoid overexertion, especially if you're hypertensive already), and paying attention to how your body feels during exercise. When you start to feel any significant physical discomfort, physical weakness, dizziness, lightheadedness, or sharp pains anywhere in your body – stop! If the discomfort persists even after you have exercised, consult with your physician.

Particularly if you're new to exercising, it's normal to feel sore muscles within the first day or two after your first exercise session. It's called delayed onset muscle soreness, and it's just your muscles' way of adapting to the new workload you're giving it. Resume exercising only after the soreness has completely gone and over time, you won't feel that anymore as your body starts to get used to exercising.

Practical Exercising Tips

Exercising isn't normal for most people – it may be the case for you. If that's the case, it can be quite challenging to start and keep a regular exercise routine. But with these practical tips, you can sustain the habit of regular exercise.

The first tip is to choose a fun exercise. Remember one of the 2 questions I posed earlier to help you choose a particular activity or exercise? If you choose a fun exercise activity, practically half the willpower battle to establish and maintain a regular exercise routine is won. Be it brisk walking with your spouse, biking with your best friend, light jogging with your kids, or swimming at the local YMCA facility, choosing a fun exercise activity will make you excited to exercise instead of feeling you have to exercise.

Another practical tip in terms of exercising for lower blood pressure is enrolling in a gym and hiring a coach or instructor. While it's not mandatory to use gym equipment, enrolling in one can motivate you by being with other people who exercise regularly. It's like the more you hang out with fitness-minded people, the higher the chances of you developing the discipline, habit and desire to exercise regularly. Plus, hiring a coach or instructor helps unload the burden of having to figure out what exercises to do and how much to do off your shoulders. All you need to think about is hauling your body to the gym and doing what the instructor tells you. It's that convenient and simple.

Do Some Resistance Training

While doing cardiovascular exercises is the best exercise for helping you lower blood pressure, consider the possibility of augmenting it with some resistance or weight training, especially if you're a bit on the heavy or plump side. Why?

When it comes to losing weight, i.e., burning off body fat, resistance training is the best way to do it. It helps you maintain – if not increase – muscle mass, which is a key determinant of metabolism or the ability to burn calories and body fat. The more muscle mass you have, the more fat and calories your body can burn on a regular basis – even while at rest.

Resistance training isn't limited to lifting weights at the gym. Many resistance training exercises can be done with a pair of light dumbbells, resistance bands, or your own body weight. And resistance training doesn't necessarily mean lifting like a power lifter or doing bodyweight exercises like the Navy SEALs. Remember, the key is to perform moderate intensity.

When you lose even just 10 pounds, you can significantly bring down your risks for hypertension or if you already are hypertensive, losing that much weight may lead to a reduction of your blood pressure by several points. Just make sure you consult your doctor before embarking on a weight or resistance training program and engage the services of a physical trainer to ensure safety.

Chapter 7: Physical Approach To Lowering Blood Pressure

The third and final part of the holistic approach to lowering your blood pressure is how you live your life. While nutrition and exercise make up bulk of the hypertension management process, it doesn't mean lifestyle has not contribution to it whatsoever. Fact is, lifestyle may be just as significant as exercising when it comes to lowering your blood pressure or minimizing your risks for hypertension. And in this final chapter, we'll take a look at practical ways you can tweak your lifestyle – if needed – to maximize the results of your anti-hypertension campaign.

The Hypertension – Smoking Link

Consider this: your blood pressure rises for several minutes as soon as you finish a cigarette or two. While I'd like to get into the excruciating details of why this is so, I won't for the sake of time and so as not to overload you with information, which may actually make your blood pressure rise. Suffice to say, it's a scientific fact that smoking contributes directly to hypertension.

Therefore, one of the most practical, common sense ways you can lower your blood pressure or to minimize your risks for hypertension is by quitting. I know it's very hard as millions of smokers have tried quitting – often times going cold turkey – and failed. But it doesn't mean quitting the habit is an exercise in futility. Truth is, many people have successfully kicked the habit away and stay nicotine-free. So you can do it too.

One way to successfully kick the habit is – unless you're already terminally ill – to avoid going cold turkey, which is the equivalent of trying to lose 100 pounds of fat by crash dieting after you've been used to binge eating for practically your whole teenage and adult life. Instead, take baby steps. Reduce the number of sticks you smoke by 1 stick per day – say for a week or two. Then as you get acclimatized to smoking 1 stick less everyday for the past week or two, reduce your smokes by another stick for another week or two, and continue reducing your daily consumption by 1 stick every week until you have completely nicked the habit.

The beauty of taking baby steps is that you build up your confidence in your ability to kick the habit and motivate yourself even more each passing week through little victories. By going for small victories instead of one big victory, you minimize your risks for being discouraged by a massive failure and instead, suffer minimal discouragements through smaller ones.

Another way to kick the habit successfully over the long term is to see where your fixation for cigarettes came from, i.e., what triggered the habit in the first place. Are you a stress smoker, a social smoker (to fit in), or is it due to an oral fixation? By knowing why you're smoking, you can kick the habit by focusing on what's causing it. Instead of focusing on the symptom, you can address what's causing the symptom, which will cut the habit for good.

Lastly, think of a very compelling reason why you want to quit smoking. Pardon me for saying this but I think living a longer and quality life should be more than enough reasons for you to kick the habit. If not, consider the people you'll be leaving behind and how devastated they'll be if you die early, e.g., spouse, kids, and parents.

Often times, people who failed at quitting don't really have a compelling reason to do so. Their reasons are so shallow so as to override the overwhelming desire to smoke. If you want to see how effective having a compelling reason is in terms of successfully persevering in the midst of great adversity, look no further than the Navy SEALs and the Marines, whose trainings aren't fit for any rational and normal human being. Despite the inhuman training programs they had to go through just to be officially counted as members of those elite forces, they were able to persevere and graduate because when they start to falter and fade, they'd ask themselves why they're doing it and often times, remembering their compelling reasons were enough to give them the second wind needed to succeed.

Relaxation

When it comes to lifestyle factors that increase the risk for hypertension or for worsening it, nothing else comes close to stress, especially the chronic or continuing kind. But temporary or occasional stress can also put you at risk for hypertension, albeit indirectly, through your coping mechanisms such as binge eating, smoking, or excessive drinking. And the best way to combat stress, which unfortunately is unavoidable, is to learn how to relax. And here are practical ways you can relax in order to reduce stress levels and eventually, bring down your blood pressure.

- *Meditation*: Research has shown that as little as a few minutes of meditation daily can help ease anxiety, primarily by altering your brain's neural pathways in ways that enable you to become more resilient to stressful situations. In other words, meditation helps strengthen your mind against the evil forces of stress! So how do you practice meditation? Simple, just sit straight on a chair – preferably with back support – and both your feet planted flat on the floor. With your eyes closed, pay close attention to your reciting a specific phrase or word – also known as mantra – that will help you feel relaxed or calm such as "Nothing can rob me of my peace", "I am in control of my emotions and I will not be anxious", or any of your favorite scripture passages from the Bible, Torah, Koran, or the particular scriptures for your faith. With one hand on your tummy, time your mantra recitation together with your breaths. And whenever thoughts come popping in, don't struggle to deny them. Instead, acknowledge them and immediately let them go. Do this for at least 5 minutes, 2 to 3 times daily throughout the day.

– **Deep Breathing:** Deep breathing is one of the best ways to slow down your heart rate and calm you down, particularly when you're feeling stressed and anxious. Notice your breathing whenever you're feeling nervous, anxious or agitated. Chances are, they're short, fast and shallow. That's why breathing mindfully can go a long way in helping you manage your stress. For a couple of times during the day, take time off from what your doing and do nothing else but just focus on your breathing for about 5 minutes. Sit up straight, close your eyes, place one hand on your tummy and take slow and deep breaths through your nose. As you take breaths, pay attention to how your tummy expands as your breathe in and how the sensation travels from your belly to your head. Breathe out slowly through your mouth and repeat for about 5 minutes.

– **Keep Your Mind On The Now**: Another way to relax in the midst of stressful situations is taking your mind off your anxiety and focusing it on the things that are happening at the moment. In meditation circles, this is called the art of mindfulness or paying attention to the smallest details of the moment. When taking a walk for example, try paying attention to how the wind feels as it brushes against the skin of your face or the sensations of your feet hitting the ground with each step. When you're able to do that, you can learn – over time – to instantly take your mind off those things that are triggering your anxiety or stress and in the process, calm down and relax.

- **_Socialize_**: No man is an island. All of us were created to enjoy the company of others, whether one person at a time or as a group. It's one of the things that give us joy and peace. Notice how it feels talking to someone while going through something very challenging and stressful – how merely talking to other people about what you're going through or what you're passionate about helps you feel much better? That's why I highly encourage you to constantly keep in touch with your friends and family – spend regular quality time with them. When you do that, you'll be able to combat the stress by enjoying more happy hormones.

- **_Get Regular Massages_**: I can go on and on about the benefits of getting regular massages in terms of managing the stresses of daily living. One of the reasons why massages help a lot in terms of relaxation is that it loosens muscles that have become tense and tight due to stress – and the usual affected muscles are the neck and the trapezius muscles, the latter being the muscles connecting your neck to your shoulders. Here's how you can loosen and relax those muscles for optimal relaxation and stress relief.

- Wrap something warm around your neck and shoulders, such as a face towel soaked in warm water (wringed so it wouldn't be dripping wet) or a couple of warm compresses for about 10 minutes. With the wraps on and your eyes closed, relax your facial and upper body muscles one at a time, i.e., face, neck, traps, shoulders, chest, and upper back. When the 10 minutes of warm wrap or compress are up, remove them from your neck and shoulders and massage away your muscle tension using a tennis ball. How?

- Lean back against a wall with the tennis ball sandwiched in between with gentle pressure such that it provides a good enough pressure on that point in your back. Gently roll the ball to different spots across your upper back while maintaining the gentle pressure all throughout, which will allow you to enjoy a good back massage all by yourself.

- *Laugh Heartily*: Did you know that a hearty laugh – you know, the kind that comes from the belly – doesn't just help you reduce your mental load but also helps reduce your body's production of cortisol, the stress hormone. Even better, it also helps you flood your brain with the opposite kind of hormones – happy ones – called endorphins, which can help lighten up your feeling. Personally, I subscribed to the Saturday Night Live (SNL) and Blue Collar TV (for Redneck jokes) YouTube channels to get my daily fix of belly laughs. You can do the same or just hang out with your funniest friends.

- *Listen To Your Favorite Music*: Ever heard of the saying that music calms a savage beast? Turns out there's a scientific basis for that statement as researches have shown that music – particularly the soothing kind, not rock and roll or gangsta rap – helps bring down anxiety, heart rate, and consequently blood pressure. With today's technology like Spotify and iTunes, it's very convenient to create a playlist of your most favorite and soothing soundtracks and for listening on your phone wherever you go for anxiety and hypertensive relief!

- *Move Around*: While it's true that a most people who run regularly enjoy what's called a "runner's high", you don't have to run in order to experience something similar. Truth is, even exercises like brisk walking and yoga can help you manage stress much better through improved relaxation via production of happy hormones that produce the same kind of high as with running. You can do something as simple as brisk walking around the block or going up several flights of stairs several times to help your brain release those happy hormones and relax your way to stress relief.

- *The Power Of Gratitude*: If two of the biggest sources of stress are discontentment and greed, then its antidote – gratitude – is one of the biggest sources of peace and relaxation. When you're perennially discontented with your life and what you have, you'll always be stressed out trying to accumulate stuff you don't have, which can be quite a lot if you're discontented and greedy. One good way to cultivate the attitude of gratefulness is keeping a journal or list of things you have that most other people in the world don't that you often take for granted like an air-conditioned room, a safe job that provides well for your and your family's needs, or as simple as 24-hour access to potable water, which millions of people in places like Africa are literally dying to have.

Regular Monitoring

The key to lowering your blood pressure or simply minimizing your risks for it is by regularly monitoring it. As I mentioned earlier, blood pressure – or hypertension for that matter – doesn't happen overnight. It will seem like so only if you haven't been looking at your blood pressure for the last few months or years. But if you make checking it a daily habit, you'll be able to nip the problem in the bud.

If you're trying to lower your blood pressure, daily monitoring will also give you valuable insight as to whether or not you're doing the right things when it comes to bringing down your blood pressure. And if based on your blood pressure measurements you're not, you can quickly make the necessary nutritional, exercise, and lifestyle adjustments to bring you back on the right path.

Conclusion

Thank you again for downloading this book!

I hope this book was able to help you to learn much about how to manage hypertension, particularly how to bring it down. You learned about the 3 key pillars (outside of medication) – diet, exercise, and lifestyle and how each interplays in affecting your blood pressure. More than that, you also learned 9 deliciously easy to prepare DASH diet recipes to help you hit the ground running when it comes to bringing down your blood pressure.

The next step is to apply what you've learned, for knowing is only half the hypertension battle. Take baby steps – don't do everything at once. Start with your diet. Each week, apply one thing you learned in the book then add another one week after week. The important thing is you start as soon as possible. Then gradually build up.

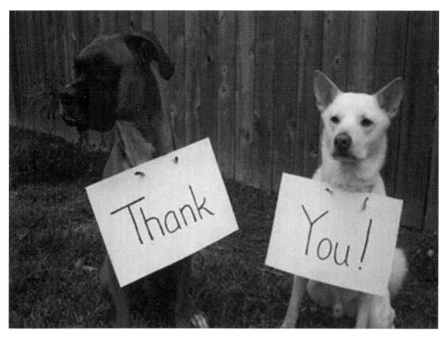

Finally, if you enjoyed this book, then I'd like to ask you for a favor, would you be kind enough to leave a review for this book on Amazon? It'd be greatly appreciated!

Click here to leave a review for this book on Amazon!

Thank you and good luck!

Made in the USA
San Bernardino, CA
04 April 2017